BLOOD TYPE O

COOKBOOK AND FOOD LIST GUIDE

Ignite your body with delicious recipes
Tailored for Fighting disease and staying
healthy

Dr. ANDY PALMER

TABLE OF CONTENTS

INTRODUCTION **9**

Blood Type O Basics **11**

Characteristics of Blood Type O 11

The science behind the Blood Type O Diet

....13

Building a Blood Type O Kitchen **15**

Stocking Blood Type O-Friendly

Ingredients 15

Kitchen Tools and Gadgets...................18

Blood Type O Food List Guide....................**23**

28-day Meal Plans for Blood Type O.........**33**

Week 1:..33

Week 2:..38

Week 3:..43

Week 4:..48

Breakfast Delights......................................**54**

Scrambled Eggs with Spinach and Turkey Sausage 54

Smoothie with Blueberries, Almond Milk, and Protein Powder 55

Omelette with Peppers, Onions, and Feta Cheese 56

Quinoa Porridge with Mixed Berries 58

Greek Yogurt Parfait with Granola and Sliced Bananas 59

Banana Oat Pancakes 60

Quinoa and Berry Breakfast Bowl 61

Green Smoothie Bowl............................. 62

Lentil Soup with Mixed Greens 64

Lunchtime Favorites....................................66

Turkey and Vegetable Stir-Fry with Brown Rice 66

Grilled Chicken Salad with Mixed Greens and Cherry Tomatoes 67

Turkey and Avocado Lettuce Wraps 68

Lentil Soup with a Side of Mixed Greens 69

Quinoa Salad with Mixed Vegetables and Grilled Chicken..............................71

Chicken Caesar Salad with Romaine Lettuce and Cherry Tomatoes..............72

Turkey Burger Lettuce Wraps with Grilled Zucchini 73

Tofu and Vegetable Stir-Fry with Brown Rice..74

Salmon and Quinoa Bowl with Steamed Broccoli......................................75

Turkey and Vegetable Wrap with Hummus..76

Dinner Creations.......................................78

Baked Cod with Lemon and Herbs, Served with Quinoa 78

Lamb Chops with Sweet Potato Wedges and Asparagus 79

Stir-fried beef with Vegetables and Brown Rice 81

Baked Halibut with Lemon-Dill Sauce... 82

Stir-fried shrimp with Broccoli and Brown 83

Baked Cod with Lemon and Herbs 84

Grilled Salmon with Lemon-Dill Sauce.. 85

Stir-fried beef with Broccoli and Brown Rice 87

Baked Chicken Thighs with Rosemary and Sweet Potato.. 88

Turkey and Vegetable Curry with Cauliflower Rice...................................... 89

Baked Cod with Tomato and Olive Relish 91

Snacks and Appetizers 93

Guacamole with Veggie Sticks 93

Hard-Boiled Eggs with Dill 94

Mixed Berry Smoothie Bowl 95

Stuffed Cherry Tomatoes with Tuna Salad 96

Hummus with Sliced Bell Peppers 97

Celery Sticks with Almond Butter 99

Sliced Turkey Roll-Ups with Avocado 99

Kale Chips with Sea Salt 100

Cucumber Rounds with Smoked Salmon 101

Seaweed Snack Rolls with Avocado ..102

Blood Type O-Friendly Beverages...........104

Green Tea with Lemon 104

Cucumber Mint Infused Water 105

Pineapple Ginger Refresher 106

Dandelion Root Tea 107

Coconut Water with Lime 108

Beetroot and Carrot Juice 108

Blackberry Basil Lemonade 109

Matcha Latte 111

Rooibos Tea with Orange 112

Carrot Ginger Zinger 113

Conclusion **114**

BONUS **118**

Grocery shopping tips 118

INTRODUCTION

The Blood Type O diet is a nutrition strategy based on the concept that an individual's blood type influences their dietary requirements. According to this theory, individuals with Blood Type O are thought to benefit from a diet reminiscent of their ancestral hunter-gatherer lifestyle. The core principles involve a focus on lean proteins, including meat and fish, while limiting grains and dairy.

Proponents of the Blood Type O diet claim that aligning dietary choices with one's blood type can lead to various health benefits. These include improved digestion, increased energy levels, and potential weight management. The diet suggests that certain foods may be less compatible with Blood Type O individuals, urging avoidance of these items to optimize health.

While anecdotal evidence supports the positive experiences of some adherents, scientific validation of the Blood Type O diet remains limited. It is essential for individuals considering this dietary approach to exercise caution, seeking guidance from healthcare professionals to ensure nutritional balance and adequacy for their unique health needs.

Chapter 1

Blood Type O Basics

Characteristics of Blood Type O

Blood Type O individuals exhibit distinctive traits that are believed to align with their ancestral roots and influence various aspects of their health and lifestyle.

Physical Traits: Blood Type O individuals are often described as having robust and sturdy physical characteristics. They are thought to inherit the qualities of their hunter-gatherer ancestors, possessing a natural athleticism and endurance. The belief is that individuals with Blood Type O may thrive in physically demanding activities, reflecting the evolutionary adaptations necessary for survival in challenging environments.

Personality Tendencies: While not universally agreed upon, some proponents of blood type personality theories suggest that Blood Type O individuals may exhibit specific personality traits. They are often associated with qualities such as being practical, goal-oriented, and decisive. However, it's crucial to approach such personality attributions with skepticism, as scientific support for blood type-based personality traits is generally lacking.

Dietary Recommendations: The Blood Type O diet is tailored to these individuals' presumed characteristics. It typically includes a focus on animal proteins, suggesting that a diet reminiscent of their ancestors can promote better health outcomes. This dietary approach proposes that certain foods may be less compatible with Blood Type O, encouraging the avoidance of specific items to optimize digestion and overall well-being.

The science behind the Blood Type O Diet

The science behind the Blood Type O diet is grounded in the belief that an individual's blood type influences their body's physiological responses to various foods. According to proponents of this theory, Blood Type O individuals are considered the original "hunter" blood type, and their dietary recommendations are designed to mirror the presumed eating habits of their ancient ancestors.

The rationale suggests that Blood Type O individuals may possess specific digestive and metabolic characteristics that make them better adapted to a diet rich in animal proteins, particularly lean meats and fish. It is proposed that certain foods, such as grains and dairy, may be less compatible with their digestive systems.

While blood-type antigens may influence some physiological processes, the connection to dietary preferences and health outcomes is not well-established. Most nutritional guidelines emphasize individual variations and overall dietary patterns rather than blood type specificity. Before adopting the Blood Type O diet, individuals are advised to consult with healthcare professionals to ensure nutritional adequacy and consider the broader body of evidence supporting general principles of healthy eating. Personalized dietary choices should be based on a comprehensive understanding of individual health needs and lifestyle factors.

Chapter 2

Building a Blood Type O Kitchen

Stocking Blood Type O-Friendly Ingredients

Stocking your kitchen with Blood Type O-friendly ingredients is essential to successfully follow the dietary recommendations tailored to this blood type.

Here's a guide to stocking your kitchen with Blood Type O-friendly ingredients:

1. **Lean Proteins:**

    - Skinless poultry (chicken, turkey)

    - Lean cuts of beef and lamb

    - Fish (especially those rich in omega-3 fatty acids, like salmon and mackerel)

15

2. **Vegetables:**
   - Leafy greens (kale, spinach, collard greens)
   - Broccoli and Brussels sprouts
   - Sweet potatoes and yams

3. **Fruits:**
   - Berries (blueberries, strawberries)
   - Cherries
   - Pineapple

4. **Beans and Legumes:**
   - Black beans
   - Lentils
   - Navy beans

5. **Healthy Fats:**
   - Olive oil
   - Flaxseed oil
   - Nuts (especially walnuts and almonds)

6. **Dairy Alternatives:**
   - Goat milk and cheese
   - Soy or almond milk (if well-tolerated)

7. **Grains:**
   - Quinoa
   - Rice (especially brown rice)
   - Ezekiel bread (sprouted grain bread)

8. **Herbs and Spices:**
   - Turmeric
   - Ginger
   - Garlic

9. **Beverages:**
   - Green tea
   - Water (hydration is crucial)
   - Red wine (in moderation)

10. **Condiments:**
    - Tamari sauce (instead of traditional soy sauce)

- Mustard
- Apple cider vinegar

Kitchen Tools and Gadgets

Here's a list of essential kitchen tools for individuals following the Blood Type O diet:

1. Sharp Knives:

   - Invest in a good set of sharp knives for slicing and chopping meats, vegetables, and fruits.

2. Cutting Board:

   - Use a separate cutting board for meats and vegetables to prevent cross-contamination.

3. Blender or Food Processor:

   - Ideal for preparing smoothies, sauces, and pureeing vegetables.

4. Grill or Grill Pan:

- Perfect for cooking lean cuts of meat and fish, enhancing flavor without added fats.

5. Steamer Basket:

- Ideal for cooking vegetables while retaining their nutritional value.

6. Baking Sheets and Roasting Pans:

- Great for roasting lean meats and vegetables in the oven.

7. Spiralizer:

- Transform vegetables into noodle-like shapes for creative, healthy dishes.

8. Wok or Stir-Fry Pan:

- Cook vegetables and proteins quickly while preserving their nutrients.

9. Digital Meat Thermometer:

  - Ensure meats are cooked to the appropriate internal temperature for safety.

10. Herb and Spice Grinder:

  - Grind fresh herbs and spices to enhance the flavor of your dishes.

11. Salad Spinner:

  - Efficiently wash and dry leafy greens for salads.

12. Measuring Cups and Spoons:

- Accurately measure ingredients for precise cooking and baking.

13. Food Storage Containers:

- Store prepped ingredients and leftovers, promoting the organization and reducing waste.

14. Mandoline Slicer:

- Achieve uniform slices for vegetables and fruits.

15. Non-Stick Cookware:

- Use non-stick pans to reduce the need for excessive cooking oils.

16. Citrus Juicer:

- Extract fresh juice from citrus fruits to add flavor to dishes.

17. Kitchen Scale:

- Measure ingredients by weight for more precise cooking and portion control.

18. Vegetable Peeler:

- Easily peel and prepare a variety of vegetables.

Chapter 3

Blood Type O Food List Guide

The Blood Type O food list is designed to cater to individuals with Blood Type O, here's a Blood Type O Food List and guide:

Proteins:

Recommended:

- Lean beef
- Lamb
- Veal
- Turkey
- Chicken
- Duck
- Game meats (venison, elk)

Limit or Avoid:

- Pork

- Bacon

- Ham

- Shellfish

Fish:

Recommended:

- Cod

- Haddock

- Mackerel

- Pickerel

- Red snapper

- Salmon

- Trout

Limit or Avoid:

- Catfish

- Caviar

- Octopus

- Clams

Dairy and Dairy Alternatives:

Recommended:

- Goat cheese

- Feta cheese

- Mozzarella

- Almond milk

- Soy milk

Limit or Avoid:

- Cow's milk

- Blue cheese

- American cheese

Vegetables:

Recommended:

- Spinach

- Kale

- Broccoli

- Brussels sprouts

- Sweet potatoes

- Onions

- Garlic

Limit or Avoid:

- Corn

- Cabbage

- Eggplant

- Potatoes

Fruits:

Recommended:

- Berries (blueberries, strawberries)

- Cherries

- Plums

- Pineapple

Limit or Avoid:

- Oranges

- Mangoes

- Cantaloupe

- Coconut

Grains:

Recommended:

- Quinoa

- Brown rice

- Sprouted grain bread

Limit or Avoid:

- Wheat

- Barley

- Corn

- Oats

Legumes:

Recommended:

- Black beans

- Lentils

- Navy beans

Limit or Avoid:

- Kidney beans

- Lima beans

Nuts and Seeds:

Recommended:

- Walnuts

- Almonds

- Flaxseeds

Limit or Avoid:

- Peanuts

- Cashews

Fats and Oils:

Recommended:

- Olive oil

- Flaxseed oil

Limit or Avoid:

- Corn oil

- Cottonseed oil

Beverages:

Recommended:

- Green tea

- Red wine (in moderation)

Limit or Avoid:

- Coffee

- Black tea

Herbs and Spices:

Recommended:

- Turmeric

- Ginger

- Garlic

Limit or Avoid:

- Cilantro

- Corn silk

Sweeteners:

Recommended:

- Agave nectar

- Maple syrup

Limit or Avoid:

- White sugar

- Corn syrup

Condiments:

Recommended:

- Tamari sauce (instead of soy sauce)

- Mustard

- Apple cider vinegar

Limit or Avoid:

- Ketchup

- Mayonnaise

Miscellaneous:

Recommended:

- Seaweed

- Tofu

Limit or Avoid:

- Processed foods

- Artificial additives

Chapter 4

28-day Meal Plans for Blood Type O

Creating a 28-day meal plan for the Blood Type O diet involves incorporating a variety of recommended foods while considering balance and nutritional adequacy. Always consult with healthcare professionals for personalized advice.

Week 1:

Day 1:

- Breakfast: Scrambled eggs with spinach and turkey sausage

- Snack: Greek yogurt with sliced strawberries

- Lunch: Grilled chicken salad with mixed greens and cherry tomatoes

- Snack: Handful of almonds

- Dinner: Baked salmon with quinoa and steamed broccoli

- Beverage: Green tea

Day 2:

- Breakfast: Smoothie with blueberries, almond milk, and protein powder

- Snack: Apple slices with almond butter

- Lunch: Turkey and avocado lettuce wraps

- Snack: Carrot and cucumber sticks with hummus

- Dinner: Stir-fried beef with vegetables and brown rice

- Beverage: Water with lemon

Day 3:

- Breakfast: Omelette with peppers, onions, and feta cheese

- Snack: Banana slices with almond butter

- Lunch: Lentil soup with a side of mixed greens

- Snack: Celery sticks with guacamole

- Dinner: Grilled lamb chops with sweet potato wedges and asparagus

- Beverage: Herbal tea

Day 4:

- Breakfast: Quinoa porridge with mixed berries

- Snack: Cherry tomatoes with mozzarella cheese

- Lunch: Tofu and vegetable stir-fry with brown rice

- Snack: Greek yogurt with a handful of walnuts

- Dinner: Baked cod with lemon and herbs, served with steamed broccoli

- Beverage: Water with mint leaves

Day 5:

- Breakfast: Greek yogurt parfait with granola and sliced bananas

- Snack: Carrot sticks with hummus

- Lunch: Chicken and vegetable curry with cauliflower rice

- Snack: Apple slices with a sprinkle of cinnamon

- Dinner: Turkey burgers with lettuce wraps and a side of grilled zucchini

- Beverage: Green tea with ginger

Day 6:

- Breakfast: Scrambled eggs with sautéed spinach and tomatoes

- Snack: Cottage cheese with pineapple chunks

- Lunch: Quinoa salad with mixed vegetables and grilled chicken

- Snack: Mixed berries (blueberries, raspberries, blackberries)

- Dinner: Stir-fried shrimp with broccoli and brown rice

- Beverage: Water with cucumber slices

Day 7:

- Breakfast: Smoothie with kale, pineapple, and coconut water

- Snack: Handful of cashews

- Lunch: Grilled steak with roasted sweet potatoes and green beans

- Snack: Sliced pear with almond butter

- Dinner: Baked halibut with lemon-dill sauce, served with quinoa

- Beverage: Herbal tea with honey

Week 2:

Day 8:

- Breakfast: Quinoa porridge with mixed berries

- Snack: Greek yogurt with a handful of almonds

- Lunch: Turkey and vegetable stir-fry with brown rice

- Snack: Apple slices with almond butter

- Dinner: Grilled salmon with lemon-dill sauce, served with steamed broccoli

- Beverage: Water with mint leaves

Day 9:

- Breakfast: Smoothie with spinach, banana, and almond milk

- Snack: Handful of walnuts

- Lunch: Chicken Caesar salad with romaine lettuce and cherry tomatoes

- Snack: Sliced cucumber with hummus

- Dinner: Beef and vegetable kebabs with quinoa

- Beverage: Green tea with ginger

Day 10:

- Breakfast: Omelette with mushrooms, onions, and feta cheese

- Snack: Banana slices with almond butter

- Lunch: Lentil soup with a side of mixed greens

- Snack: Celery sticks with guacamole

- Dinner: Grilled lamb chops with sweet potato wedges and asparagus

- Beverage: Water with lemon

Day 11:

- Breakfast: Greek yogurt parfait with granola and mixed berries

- Snack: Carrot sticks with hummus

- Lunch: Tofu and vegetable stir-fry with brown rice

- Snack: Apple slices with a sprinkle of
  cinnamon

- Dinner: Baked cod with lemon and
  herbs, served with quinoa

- Beverage: Herbal tea

Day 12:

- Breakfast: Scrambled eggs with
  sautéed spinach and tomatoes

- Snack: Cottage cheese with
  pineapple chunks

- Lunch: Quinoa salad with mixed
  vegetables and grilled chicken

- Snack: Mixed berries (blueberries,
  raspberries, blackberries)

- Dinner: Stir-fried shrimp with broccoli
  and brown rice

- Beverage: Water with cucumber slices

Day 13:

- Breakfast: Smoothie with kale, pineapple, and coconut water

- Snack: Handful of cashews

- Lunch: Grilled steak with roasted sweet potatoes and green beans

- Snack: Sliced pear with almond butter

- Dinner: Baked halibut with lemon-dill sauce, served with steamed asparagus

- Beverage: Water with mint leaves

Day 14:

- Breakfast: Quinoa porridge with sliced bananas and a drizzle of honey

- Snack: Greek yogurt with a handful of walnuts

- Lunch: Turkey and avocado lettuce wraps

- Snack: Carrot and cucumber sticks with hummus

- Dinner: Stir-fried beef with broccoli and brown rice

- Beverage: Green tea with ginger

Week 3:

Day 15:

- Breakfast: Scrambled eggs with spinach and turkey sausage

- Snack: Greek yogurt with mixed berries

- Lunch: Grilled chicken salad with mixed greens and cherry tomatoes

- Snack: Handful of almonds

- Dinner: Baked salmon with quinoa and steamed broccoli

- Beverage: Green tea

Day 16:

- Breakfast: Smoothie with blueberries, almond milk, and protein powder

- Snack: Apple slices with almond butter

- Lunch: Turkey and avocado lettuce wraps

- Snack: Carrot and cucumber sticks with hummus

- Dinner: Stir-fried beef with vegetables and brown rice

- Beverage: Water with lemon

Day 17:

- Breakfast: Omelette with peppers, onions, and feta cheese

- Snack: Banana slices with almond butter

- Lunch: Lentil soup with a side of mixed greens

- Snack: Celery sticks with guacamole

- Dinner: Grilled lamb chops with sweet potato wedges and asparagus

- Beverage: Herbal tea

Day 18:

- Breakfast: Quinoa porridge with mixed berries

- Snack: Cherry tomatoes with mozzarella cheese

- Lunch: Tofu and vegetable stir-fry with brown rice

- Snack: Greek yogurt with a handful of walnuts

- Dinner: Baked cod with lemon and herbs, served with steamed broccoli

- Beverage: Water with mint leaves

Day 19:

- Breakfast: Greek yogurt parfait with granola and sliced bananas

- Snack: Carrot sticks with hummus

- Lunch: Chicken and vegetable curry with cauliflower rice

- Snack: Apple slices with a sprinkle of cinnamon

- Dinner: Turkey burgers with lettuce wraps and a side of grilled zucchini

- Beverage: Green tea with ginger

Day 20:

- Breakfast: Scrambled eggs with sautéed spinach and tomatoes

- Snack: Cottage cheese with pineapple chunks

- Lunch: Quinoa salad with mixed vegetables and grilled chicken

- Snack: Mixed berries (blueberries, raspberries, blackberries)

- Dinner: Stir-fried shrimp with broccoli and brown rice

- Beverage: Water with cucumber slices

Day 21:

- Breakfast: Smoothie with kale, pineapple, and coconut water

- Snack: Handful of cashews

- Lunch: Grilled steak with roasted sweet potatoes and green beans

- Snack: Sliced pear with almond butter

- Dinner: Baked halibut with lemon-dill sauce, served with quinoa

- Beverage: Herbal tea with honey

Week 4:

Day 22:

- Breakfast: Quinoa porridge with mixed berries

- Snack: Greek yogurt with a handful of almonds

- Lunch: Turkey and vegetable stir-fry with brown rice

- Snack: Apple slices with almond butter

- Dinner: Grilled salmon with lemon-dill sauce, served with steamed broccoli

- Beverage: Green tea

Day 23:

- Breakfast: Smoothie with blueberries, almond milk, and protein powder

- Snack: Apple slices with almond butter

- Lunch: Turkey and avocado lettuce wraps

- Snack: Carrot and cucumber sticks with hummus

- Dinner: Stir-fried beef with vegetables and brown rice

- Beverage: Water with lemon

Day 24:

- Breakfast: Omelette with peppers, onions, and feta cheese

- Snack: Banana slices with almond butter

- Lunch: Lentil soup with a side of mixed greens

- Snack: Celery sticks with guacamole

- Dinner: Grilled lamb chops with sweet potato wedges and asparagus

- Beverage: Herbal tea

Day 25:

- Breakfast: Quinoa porridge with mixed berries

- Snack: Cherry tomatoes with mozzarella cheese

- Lunch: Tofu and vegetable stir-fry with brown rice

- Snack: Greek yogurt with a handful of walnuts

- Dinner: Baked cod with lemon and herbs, served with steamed broccoli

- Beverage: Water with mint leaves

Day 26:

- Breakfast: Greek yogurt parfait with granola and sliced bananas

- Snack: Carrot sticks with hummus

- Lunch: Chicken and vegetable curry with cauliflower rice

- Snack: Apple slices with a sprinkle of cinnamon

- Dinner: Turkey burgers with lettuce wraps and a side of grilled zucchini

- Beverage: Green tea with ginger

Day 27:

- Breakfast: Scrambled eggs with sautéed spinach and tomatoes

- Snack: Cottage cheese with pineapple chunks

- Lunch: Quinoa salad with mixed vegetables and grilled chicken

- Snack: Mixed berries (blueberries, raspberries, blackberries)

- Dinner: Stir-fried shrimp with broccoli and brown rice

- Beverage: Water with cucumber slices

Day 28:

- Breakfast: Smoothie with kale, pineapple, and coconut water

- Snack: Handful of cashews

- Lunch: Grilled steak with roasted sweet potatoes and green beans

- Snack: Sliced pear with almond butter

- Dinner: Baked halibut with lemon-dill sauce, served with quinoa

- Beverage: Herbal tea with honey

Chapter 5

Breakfast Delights

Scrambled Eggs with Spinach and Turkey Sausage

Ingredients:

- 2 large eggs

- Handful of fresh spinach

- Lean turkey sausage, cooked

- Olive oil

- Salt and pepper to taste

Instructions:

1. In a skillet, heat olive oil over medium heat.

2. Add spinach and cook until wilted.

3. Whisk eggs and pour them into the skillet.

4. Add cooked turkey sausage and scramble until eggs are cooked.

5. Season with salt and pepper.

Nutritional Information (Approx.):

- Calories: 300

- Protein: 25g

- Fat: 18g

- Carbohydrates: 7g

Smoothie with Blueberries, Almond Milk, and Protein Powder

Ingredients:

- 1 cup blueberries

- 1 cup almond milk

- 1 scoop protein powder

- Ice cubes (optional)

Instructions:

1. Blend blueberries, almond milk, and protein powder until smooth.

2. Add ice cubes if desired and blend again.

Nutritional Information (Approx.):

- Calories: 220

- Protein: 20g

- Fat: 5g

- Carbohydrates: 25g

Omelette with Peppers, Onions, and Feta Cheese

Ingredients:

- 3 large eggs

- Red and green bell peppers, diced

- Onion, diced

- Feta cheese

- Olive oil

- Salt and pepper to taste

Instructions:

1. Whisk eggs in a bowl.

2. In a skillet, sauté peppers and onions in olive oil until tender.

3. Pour whisked eggs over the veggies.

4. Add crumbled feta cheese.

5. Cook until the eggs are set, folding the omelette in half.

Nutritional Information (Approx.):

- Calories: 350

- Protein: 20g

- Fat: 25g

- Carbohydrates: 10g

Quinoa Porridge with Mixed Berries

Ingredients:

- 1/2 cup quinoa, cooked

- Mixed berries (blueberries, strawberries)

- Almond milk

- Honey or maple syrup (optional)

Instructions:

1. Cook quinoa according to package instructions.

2. Top with mixed berries.

3. Pour almond milk over the quinoa and berries.

4. Drizzle with honey or maple syrup if desired.

Nutritional Information (Approx.):

- Calories: 300

- Protein: 10g

- Fat: 5g

- Carbohydrates: 55g

Greek Yogurt Parfait with Granola and Sliced Bananas

Ingredients:

- Greek yogurt

- Granola

- Sliced bananas

- Honey

Instructions:

1. In a glass, layer Greek yogurt, granola, and sliced bananas.

2. Repeat layers.

3. Drizzle honey on top.

Nutritional Information (Approx.):

- Calories: 400

- Protein: 20g

- Fat: 10g

- Carbohydrates: 60g

Banana Oat Pancakes

Ingredients:

- 1 ripe banana, mashed

- 1/2 cup rolled oats

- 2 eggs

- Cinnamon (optional)

Instructions:

1. Mix mashed banana, rolled oats, and eggs in a bowl.

2. Heat a skillet and pour small portions of the mixture.

3. Cook until the edges are golden brown, then flip.

4. Sprinkle with cinnamon if desired.

Nutritional Information (Approx.):

- Calories: 300

- Protein: 15g

- Fat: 10g

- Carbohydrates: 40g

Quinoa and Berry Breakfast Bowl

Ingredients:

- 1/2 cup cooked quinoa

- Mixed berries (strawberries, raspberries, blackberries)

- Almond butter

- Chia seeds

Instructions:

1. In a bowl, combine quinoa and mixed berries.

2. Drizzle with almond butter.

3. Sprinkle chia seeds on top.

Nutritional Information (Approx.):

- Calories: 350

- Protein: 12g

- Fat: 15g

- Carbohydrates: 45g

Green Smoothie Bowl

Ingredients:

- 1 cup spinach

- 1/2 avocado

- 1/2 cup pineapple chunks

- Almond milk

- Chia seeds

Instructions:

1. Blend spinach, avocado, pineapple, and almond milk until smooth.

2. Pour into a bowl.

3. Top with chia seeds.

Nutritional Information (Approx.):

- Calories: 250

- Protein: 8g

- Fat: 15g

- Carbohydrates: 30g

Lentil Soup with Mixed Greens

Ingredients:

- Green or brown lentils

- Mixed greens (spinach, kale)

- Onion, diced

- Garlic, minced

- Vegetable broth

Instructions:

1. Cook lentils according to package instructions.

2. Sauté onions and garlic in a pot.

3. Add cooked lentils and vegetable broth.

4. Add mixed greens and simmer until greens are wilted.

Nutritional Information (Approx.):

- Calories: 300

- Protein: 18g

- Fat: 5g

- Carbohydrates: 50g

Chapter 6

Lunchtime Favorites

Turkey and Vegetable Stir-Fry with Brown Rice

Ingredients:

- Sliced turkey breast

- Mixed vegetables (bell peppers, broccoli, carrots)

- Tamari sauce (or soy sauce)

- Brown rice, cooked

Instructions:

1. Stir-fry turkey slices and vegetables in a wok.

2. Add tamari sauce for flavor.

3. Serve over cooked brown rice.

Nutritional Information (Approx.):

- Calories: 350

- Protein: 25g

- Fat: 10g

- Carbohydrates: 40g

Grilled Chicken Salad with Mixed Greens and Cherry Tomatoes

Ingredients:

- Grilled chicken breast, sliced

- Mixed greens (spinach, kale, arugula)

- Cherry tomatoes, halved

- Olive oil and balsamic vinegar dressing

Instructions:

1. Arrange mixed greens on a plate.

2. Top with grilled chicken slices and cherry tomatoes.

3. Drizzle with olive oil and balsamic vinegar dressing.

Nutritional Information (Approx.):

- Calories: 400

- Protein: 30g

- Fat: 15g

- Carbohydrates: 25g

Turkey and Avocado Lettuce Wraps

Ingredients:

- Sliced turkey breast

- Romaine lettuce leaves

- Avocado, sliced

- Tomato, sliced

Instructions:

1. Lay turkey slices on lettuce leaves.

2. Add slices of avocado and tomato.

3. Wrap and enjoy.

Nutritional Information (Approx.):

- Calories: 280

- Protein: 25g

- Fat: 15g

- Carbohydrates: 10g

Lentil Soup with a Side of Mixed Greens

Ingredients:

- Green or brown lentils

- Mixed greens (spinach, kale)

- Onion, diced

- Garlic, minced

- Vegetable broth

Instructions:

1. Cook lentils according to package instructions.

2. Sauté onions and garlic in a pot.

3. Add cooked lentils and vegetable broth.

4. Add mixed greens and simmer until greens are wilted.

Nutritional Information (Approx.):

- Calories: 300

- Protein: 18g

- Fat: 5g

- Carbohydrates: 50g

Quinoa Salad with Mixed Vegetables and Grilled Chicken

Ingredients:

- Cooked quinoa

- Mixed vegetables (bell peppers, cucumber, cherry tomatoes)

- Grilled chicken breast, sliced

- Olive oil and balsamic vinegar dressing

Instructions:

1. Combine quinoa, mixed vegetables, and grilled chicken in a bowl.

2. Drizzle with olive oil and balsamic vinegar dressing.

Nutritional Information (Approx.):

- Calories: 400

- Protein: 25g

- Fat: 15g

- Carbohydrates: 40g

Chicken Caesar Salad with Romaine Lettuce and Cherry Tomatoes

Ingredients:

- Grilled chicken breast, sliced

- Romaine lettuce, chopped

- Cherry tomatoes, halved

- Caesar dressing (watch for compliance)

Instructions:

1. Combine chopped romaine lettuce, grilled chicken, and cherry tomatoes in a bowl.

2. Toss with Caesar dressing.

Nutritional Information (Approx.):

- Calories: 350

- Protein: 30g

- Fat: 20g

- Carbohydrates: 15g

Turkey Burger Lettuce Wraps with Grilled Zucchini

Ingredients:

- Turkey burger patties

- Romaine lettuce leaves

- Tomato, sliced

- Grilled zucchini slices

Instructions:

1. Grill turkey burger patties until fully cooked.

2. Place each patty on a romaine
   lettuce leaf.

3. Top with sliced tomatoes and grilled
   zucchini.

Nutritional Information (Approx.):

- Calories: 320

- Protein: 30g

- Fat: 15g

- Carbohydrates: 15g

Tofu and Vegetable Stir-Fry with Brown Rice

Ingredients:

- Firm tofu, cubed

- Mixed vegetables (broccoli, bell peppers, snap peas)

- Tamari sauce (or soy sauce)

- Brown rice, cooked

Instructions:

1. Stir-fry tofu and mixed vegetables in a wok.

2. Add tamari sauce for flavor.

3. Serve over cooked brown rice.

Nutritional Information (Approx.):

- Calories: 300

- Protein: 20g

- Fat: 12g

- Carbohydrates: 40g

Salmon and Quinoa Bowl with Steamed Broccoli

Ingredients:

- Baked or grilled salmon fillet

- Quinoa, cooked

- Steamed broccoli florets

- Lemon wedges

Instructions:

1. Place cooked quinoa in a bowl.

2. Top with salmon fillet and steamed broccoli.

3. Garnish with lemon wedges.

Nutritional Information (Approx.):

- Calories: 380

- Protein: 30g

- Fat: 18g

- Carbohydrates: 25g

Turkey and Vegetable Wrap with Hummus

Ingredients:

- Sliced turkey breast

- Whole-grain wrap

- Mixed vegetables (bell peppers, cucumber, lettuce)

- Hummus

Instructions:

1. Spread hummus on a whole-grain wrap.

2. Layer with sliced turkey and mixed vegetables.

3. Roll into a wrap and slice.

Nutritional Information (Approx.):

- Calories: 350

- Protein: 25g

- Fat: 12g

- Carbohydrates: 40g

Chapter 7

Dinner Creations

Baked Cod with Lemon and Herbs, Served with Quinoa

Ingredients:

- Cod fillets

- Lemon slices

- Fresh herbs (parsley, dill)

- Olive oil

- Salt and pepper

- Quinoa, cooked

Instructions:

1. Place cod fillets on a baking sheet.

2. Top with lemon slices and fresh herbs.

3. Drizzle with olive oil, salt, and pepper.

4. Bake until fish flakes easily with a fork.

5. Serve with cooked quinoa.

Nutritional Information (Approx.):

- Calories: 350

- Protein: 30g

- Fat: 10g

- Carbohydrates: 30g

Lamb Chops with Sweet Potato Wedges and Asparagus

Ingredients:

- Grilled lamb chops

- Sweet potato wedges

- Asparagus spears

- Olive oil

- Salt and pepper

Instructions:

1. Grill lamb chops to the desired doneness.

2. Toss sweet potato wedges and asparagus in olive oil, salt, and pepper.

3. Roast in the oven until tender.

Nutritional Information (Approx.):

- Calories: 400

- Protein: 25g

- Fat: 20g

- Carbohydrates: 30g

Stir-fried beef with Vegetables and Brown Rice

Ingredients:

- Lean beef strips

- Mixed vegetables (bell peppers, broccoli, carrots)

- Tamari sauce (or soy sauce)

- Brown rice, cooked

Instructions:

1. Stir-fry beef and vegetables in a wok.

2. Add tamari sauce for flavor.

3. Serve over cooked brown rice.

Nutritional Information (Approx.):

- Calories: 350

- Protein: 25g

- Fat: 10g

- Carbohydrates: 40g

Baked Halibut with Lemon-Dill Sauce

Ingredients:

- Halibut fillets

- Lemon juice

- Fresh dill, chopped

- Olive oil

- Salt and pepper

Instructions:

1. Place halibut fillets on a baking sheet.

2. Drizzle with lemon juice and olive oil.

3. Sprinkle with fresh dill, salt, and pepper.

4. Bake until fish flakes easily with a fork.

Nutritional Information (Approx.):

- Calories: 280

- Protein: 35g

- Fat: 10g

- Carbohydrates: 2g

Stir-fried shrimp with Broccoli and Brown Rice

Ingredients:

- Shrimp, peeled and deveined

- Broccoli florets

- Garlic, minced

- Tamari sauce (or soy sauce)

- Brown rice, cooked

Instructions:

1. Stir-fry shrimp and broccoli in a pan.

2. Add minced garlic and tamari sauce.

3. Serve over cooked brown rice.

Nutritional Information (Approx.):

- Calories: 320

- Protein: 30g

- Fat: 5g

- Carbohydrates: 40g

Baked Cod with Lemon and Herbs

Ingredients:

- Cod fillets

- Lemon slices

- Fresh herbs (parsley, dill)

- Olive oil

- Salt and pepper

Instructions:

1. Place cod fillets on a baking sheet.

2. Top with lemon slices and fresh herbs.

3. Drizzle with olive oil.

4. Bake until fish flakes easily with a fork.

Nutritional Information (Approx.):

- Calories: 250

- Protein: 30g

- Fat: 10g

- Carbohydrates: 1g

Grilled Salmon with Lemon-Dill Sauce

Ingredients:

- Salmon fillets

- Lemon juice

- Fresh dill, chopped

- Olive oil

- Salt and pepper

Instructions:

1. Place salmon fillets on a grill or in the oven.

2. Drizzle with lemon juice and olive oil.

3. Sprinkle with fresh dill, salt, and pepper.

4. Cook until fish flakes easily with a fork.

Nutritional Information (Approx.):

- Calories: 300

- Protein: 30g

- Fat: 18g

- Carbohydrates: 1g

Stir-fried beef with Broccoli and Brown Rice

Ingredients:

- Lean beef strips

- Broccoli florets

- Garlic, minced

- Tamari sauce (or soy sauce)

- Brown rice, cooked

Instructions:

1. Stir-fry beef and broccoli in a wok.

2. Add minced garlic and tamari sauce.

3. Serve over cooked brown rice.

Nutritional Information (Approx.):

- Calories: 350

- Protein: 25g

- Fat: 10g

- Carbohydrates: 40g

Baked Chicken Thighs with Rosemary and Sweet Potato

Ingredients:

- Chicken thighs, bone-in

- Fresh rosemary, chopped

- Sweet potatoes, diced

- Olive oil

- Salt and pepper

Instructions:

1. Rub chicken thighs with chopped rosemary, olive oil, salt, and pepper.

2. Place on a baking sheet.

3. Toss sweet potato cubes in olive oil, salt, and pepper, and place on the same sheet.

4. Bake until chicken is cooked through and sweet potatoes are tender.

Nutritional Information (Approx.):

- Calories: 380

- Protein: 30g

- Fat: 20g

- Carbohydrates: 25g

Turkey and Vegetable Curry with Cauliflower Rice

Ingredients:

- Ground turkey

- Mixed vegetables (bell peppers, carrots, peas)

- Curry sauce (watch for compliance)

- Cauliflower rice

Instructions:

1. Cook ground turkey and mixed vegetables in a pan.

2. Add curry sauce and simmer until vegetables are tender.

3. Serve over cauliflower rice.

Nutritional Information (Approx.):

- Calories: 320

- Protein: 30g

- Fat: 15g

- Carbohydrates: 20g

Baked Cod with Tomato and Olive Relish

Ingredients:

- Cod fillets

- Cherry tomatoes, halved

- Kalamata olives, sliced

- Fresh basil, chopped

- Olive oil

- Garlic, minced

Instructions:

1. Place cod fillets on a baking sheet.

2. Mix tomatoes, olives, basil, olive oil, and minced garlic in a bowl.

3. Spoon the mixture over the cod.

4. Bake until fish flakes easily with a fork.

Nutritional Information (Approx.):

- Calories: 280

- Protein: 30g

- Fat: 15g

- Carbohydrates: 5g

Chapter 8

Snacks and Appetizers

Guacamole with Veggie Sticks

Ingredients:

- Avocado

- Tomato, diced

- Onion, finely chopped

- Lime juice

- Garlic, minced

- Bell pepper and cucumber sticks

Instructions:

1. Mash the avocado and mix with diced tomato, chopped onion, lime juice, and minced garlic.

2. Serve with bell pepper and cucumber sticks for dipping.

Nutritional Information (Approx.):

- Calories: 150

- Protein: 2g

- Fat: 12g

- Carbohydrates: 10g

Hard-Boiled Eggs with Dill

Ingredients:

- Hard-boiled eggs

- Fresh dill, chopped

- Salt and pepper

Instructions:

1. Slice hard-boiled eggs.

2. Sprinkle with chopped fresh dill, salt, and pepper.

Nutritional Information (Approx.):

- Calories: 80

- Protein: 6g

- Fat: 5g

- Carbohydrates: 1g

Mixed Berry Smoothie Bowl

Ingredients:

- Mixed berries (blueberries, strawberries)

- Greek yogurt

- Almond butter

- Chia seeds

Instructions:

1. Blend mixed berries, Greek yogurt, and almond butter until smooth.

2. Pour into a bowl and top with chia seeds.

Nutritional Information (Approx.):

- Calories: 200

- Protein: 10g

- Fat: 8g

- Carbohydrates: 25g

Stuffed Cherry Tomatoes with Tuna Salad

Ingredients:

- Cherry tomatoes

- Canned tuna, drained

- Greek yogurt

- Dill, chopped

- Celery, finely chopped

Instructions:

1. Cut a small slice off the top of each cherry tomato and scoop out the seeds.

2. In a bowl, mix tuna, Greek yogurt, dill, and celery.

3. Stuff cherry tomatoes with tuna salad.

Nutritional Information (Approx.):

- Calories: 100

- Protein: 12g

- Fat: 5g

- Carbohydrates: 3g

Hummus with Sliced Bell Peppers

Ingredients:

- Chickpeas

- Tahini

- Olive oil

- Lemon juice

- Garlic, minced

- Bell pepper strips

Instructions:

1. Blend chickpeas, tahini, olive oil, lemon juice, and minced garlic until smooth.

2. Serve with sliced bell peppers for dipping.

Nutritional Information (Approx.):

- Calories: 180

- Protein: 6g

- Fat: 12g

- Carbohydrates: 15g

Celery Sticks with Almond Butter

Ingredients:

- Celery sticks

- Almond butter

Instructions:

1. Spread almond butter on celery sticks.

Nutritional Information (Approx.):

- Calories: 100

- Protein: 4g

- Fat: 8g

- Carbohydrates: 4g

Sliced Turkey Roll-Ups with Avocado

Ingredients:

- Sliced turkey breast

- Avocado, sliced

- Mustard (watch for compliance)

Instructions:

1. Lay turkey slices flat.

2. Add avocado slices and a touch of mustard.

3. Roll up and secure with toothpicks.

Nutritional Information (Approx.):

- Calories: 120

- Protein: 15g

- Fat: 6g

- Carbohydrates: 2g

Kale Chips with Sea Salt

Ingredients:

- Fresh kale, torn into pieces

- Olive oil

- Sea salt

Instructions:

1. Toss kale with olive oil and sprinkle with sea salt.

2. Bake until crisp.

Nutritional Information (Approx.):

- Calories: 80

- Protein: 3g

- Fat: 5g

- Carbohydrates: 8g

Cucumber Rounds with Smoked Salmon

Ingredients:

- Cucumber slices

- Smoked salmon

- Cream cheese (watch for compliance)

Instructions:

1. Spread a thin layer of cream cheese on cucumber slices.

2. Top with smoked salmon.

Nutritional Information (Approx.):

- Calories: 150

- Protein: 15g

- Fat: 8g

- Carbohydrates: 5g

Seaweed Snack Rolls with Avocado

Ingredients:

- Seaweed snack sheets

- Avocado, sliced

Instructions:

1. Lay seaweed sheets flat.

2. Place avocado slices on one end
    and roll up.

Nutritional Information (Approx.):

- Calories: 100

- Protein: 2g

- Fat: 8g

- Carbohydrates: 6g

Chapter 9

Blood Type O-Friendly Beverages

Green Tea with Lemon

Ingredients:

- Green tea bags

- Hot water

- Lemon slices

Instructions:

1. Steep green tea bags in hot water.

2. Add lemon slices for flavor.

Nutritional Information (Approx.):

- Calories: 0

- Protein: 0g

- Fat: 0g

- Carbohydrates: 0g

Cucumber Mint Infused Water

Ingredients:

- Cucumber slices

- Fresh mint leaves

- Water

Instructions:

1. Combine cucumber slices and fresh mint leaves in water.

2. Allow to infuse in the refrigerator.

Nutritional Information (Approx.):

- Calories: 0

- Protein: 0g

- Fat: 0g

- Carbohydrates: 0g

Pineapple Ginger Refresher

Ingredients:

- Pineapple chunks

- Fresh ginger, grated

- Sparkling water

Instructions:

1. Muddle pineapple chunks and grated ginger.

2. Mix with sparkling water.

Nutritional Information (Approx.):

- Calories: 60

- Protein: 1g

- Fat: 0g

- Carbohydrates: 15g

Dandelion Root Tea

Ingredients:

- Dandelion root tea bags

- Hot water

- Lemon wedge (optional)

Instructions:

1. Steep dandelion root tea bags in hot water.

2. Add a lemon wedge for extra flavor.

Nutritional Information (Approx.):

- Calories: 0

- Protein: 0g

- Fat: 0g

- Carbohydrates: 0g

Coconut Water with Lime

Ingredients:

- Coconut water

- Lime juice

Instructions:

1. Mix coconut water with freshly squeezed lime juice.

Nutritional Information (Approx.):

- Calories: 40

- Protein: 1g

- Fat: 0g

- Carbohydrates: 10g

Beetroot and Carrot Juice

Ingredients:

- Beetroots, peeled and chopped

- Carrots, peeled and chopped

- Ginger, grated

- Water

Instructions:

1. Juice beetroots, carrots, and ginger.

2. Dilute with water as desired.

Nutritional Information (Approx.):

- Calories: 80

- Protein: 2g

- Fat: 0g

- Carbohydrates: 20g

Blackberry Basil Lemonade

Ingredients:

- Blackberries

- Fresh basil leaves

- Lemon juice

- Water

- Stevia (optional)

Instructions:

1. Muddle blackberries and fresh basil in lemon juice.

2. Mix with water and sweeten with stevia if desired.

Nutritional Information (Approx.):

- Calories: 40

- Protein: 1g

- Fat: 0g

- Carbohydrates: 10g

Matcha Latte

Ingredients:

- Matcha powder

- Almond milk

- Honey (optional)

Instructions:

1. Whisk matcha powder with warm almond milk.

2. Sweeten with honey if desired.

Nutritional Information (Approx.):

- Calories: 50

- Protein: 2g

- Fat: 2g

- Carbohydrates: 8g

Rooibos Tea with Orange

Ingredients:

- Rooibos tea bags

- Hot water

- Orange slices

Instructions:

1. Steep rooibos tea bags in hot water.

2. Add orange slices for a citrusy twist.

Nutritional Information (Approx.):

- Calories: 0

- Protein: 0g

- Fat: 0g

- Carbohydrates: 0g

Carrot Ginger Zinger

Ingredients:

- Carrots, peeled and chopped

- Ginger, grated

- Apple, cored and chopped

- Water

Instructions:

1. Juice carrots, ginger, and apple.

2. Dilute with water as desired.

Nutritional Information (Approx.):

- Calories: 70

- Protein: 1g

- Fat: 0g

- Carbohydrates: 18g

Chapter 10

Conclusion

In conclusion, the Blood Type O Cookbook and Food List Guide is a comprehensive resource designed to empower individuals with Blood Type O by providing a tailored approach to nutrition. Through a detailed exploration of the Blood Type O diet principles, this guide elucidates the unique characteristics, health considerations, and science behind the dietary choices for individuals with Blood Type O.

By delving into the distinctive traits and tendencies associated with Blood Type O, the guide offers valuable insights into the specific foods that are beneficial and those that are best avoided. This personalized approach extends beyond general nutritional guidelines, taking into account the genetic and evolutionary factors that influence the dietary needs of individuals with Blood Type O.

The incorporation of a science-based perspective enhances the credibility of the guide, providing readers with a deeper understanding of how the Blood Type O diet aligns with biological and metabolic factors. The guide empowers individuals to make informed choices that resonate with their unique physiological makeup, fostering overall well-being.

The practical aspect of the guide extends to everyday life, with detailed sections on stocking Blood Type O-friendly ingredients and essential kitchen tools. This hands-on approach ensures that individuals can seamlessly integrate the principles of the Blood Type O diet into their culinary routines, making healthy eating a sustainable and enjoyable lifestyle.

The meticulously curated 28-day meal plans, encompassing breakfast, lunch, dinner, snacks, and beverages, further enrich the guide by providing practical examples of how to structure a Blood Type O-friendly diet. These meal plans not only cater to nutritional needs but also offer a diverse and delectable array of recipes that cater to the taste buds of individuals with Blood Type O.

In essence, the Blood Type O Cookbook and Food List Guide is more than just a collection of recipes; it's a holistic approach to nutrition that recognizes the uniqueness of each individual. By embracing the principles outlined in this guide, individuals with Blood Type O can embark on a journey towards improved health, vitality, and a harmonious relationship with food. Whether one is seeking to enhance energy levels, manage weight, or promote overall wellness, the Blood Type O Cookbook and Food List Guide serves as a valuable companion on the path to optimal health through personalized nutrition.

BONUS

Grocery shopping tips

Navigating the grocery store with the specific dietary considerations of the Blood Type O diet requires thoughtful planning and informed choices. Here's an extensive and elaborate set of grocery shopping tips tailored to the Blood Type O diet:

1. **Create a Detailed Shopping List:**

• Begin by planning your meals for the week and create a detailed shopping list based on the Blood Type O food recommendations.

• Categorize items into sections like produce, proteins, grains, and condiments to streamline your shopping experience.

2. **Prioritize Fresh, Whole Foods:**

• Focus on fresh, whole foods such as lean meats, fish, poultry, fruits, and vegetables.

- Choose organic options when possible, especially for items listed in the "beneficial" category for Blood Type O.

3. **Explore the Produce Section:**

- Load up on beneficial vegetables like kale, spinach, broccoli, and sweet potatoes.

- Opt for fruits that align with the Blood Type O diet, such as berries, cherries, and plums.

4. **Select Lean Proteins:**

- Prioritize lean proteins such as turkey, lamb, and fish like cod and mackerel.

- Consider incorporating organ meats like liver, as they are often recommended for Blood Type O.

5. **Include Healthy Fats:**

- Choose healthy fats like olive oil, flaxseed oil, and nut butter in moderation.

- Avocados and nuts like walnuts and almonds can be excellent sources of healthy fats.

6. **Dairy and Alternatives:**

- For those who tolerate dairy well, opt for beneficial options like goat or sheep's milk products.

- Non-dairy alternatives like almond or rice milk can also be considered.

7. **Grains and Legumes:**

- Select grains such as quinoa, rice, and oats, which are generally well-tolerated.

- Legumes like lentils and black-eyed peas can be included in moderation.

8. **Mindful Beverage Choices:**

- Choose beverages in alignment with the Blood Type O diet, such as green tea, herbal teas, and plenty of water.

- Minimize or avoid caffeine, especially if it is recommended for Blood Type O.

9. **Check Labels for Avoided Ingredients:**

- Scrutinize food labels for ingredients that are best avoided, such as certain additives, preservatives, and artificial colorings.

- Be aware of hidden ingredients in processed foods that may not align with the Blood Type O diet.

10. **Fresh Herbs and Spices:**

- Enhance the flavor of your dishes with fresh herbs and spices, such as ginger, turmeric, and parsley.

- Use beneficial seasonings to add depth to your meals without compromising on dietary guidelines.

11. **Limit Processed and Refined Foods:**

- Minimize the purchase of processed and refined foods, as they often contain ingredients that may not be suitable for Blood Type O.

12. **Bulk Buying for Staples:**

- Consider buying certain staples like grains, nuts, and seeds in bulk to save money and reduce packaging waste.

13. **Be Open to Variety:**

- Embrace variety in your diet by trying different fruits, vegetables, and proteins that are beneficial for Blood Type O.

14. **Stay Organized and Efficient:**

- Arrange your shopping list in the order of the store layout to save time and minimize the chances of impulse purchases.

15. **Keep an Eye on Portion Sizes:**

- Be mindful of portion sizes to ensure that you're consuming a balanced and satisfying diet while adhering to Blood Type O guidelines.

Remember, individual tolerance to certain foods can vary, so it's essential to pay attention to how your body responds to different items. Regularly reassess your grocery list based on your health goals and any feedback from your body. With these tips, grocery shopping for the Blood Type O diet can be a purposeful and enjoyable experience.